# Part 2.
# Before you start

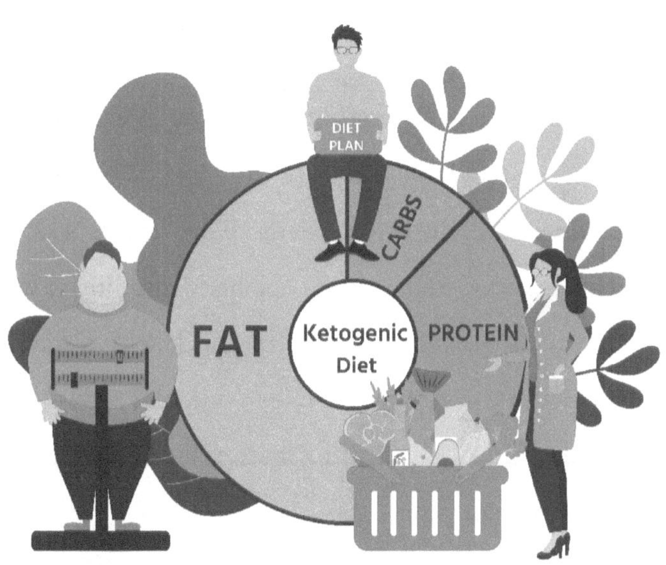

# Common mistakes of all beginners

You must have come across when surfing social media platforms about celebrities and famous figures who followed certain diets and lifestyle programs. It can make you consider following the same method as well after seeing photos of the magnificent results. That's when your first mistakes happen.

Before we jump into any diet of any sorts we must first understand that not all body types are the same. We all have different metabolism rates and nutrition needs. That means not because a certain diet worked for your favorite celebrity meaning it will work as perfectly for you as well. It is crucial to check with a nutritionist or doctor before taking a drastic turn in your diet. Even though the internet provides almost all the information we need to know but not all information is accurate.

As we have already described above, the keto diet has not only significant advantages but also real disadvantages and risks. So to make sure that it works correctly you must be fully aware of how it affects the body and its side effects.

Let's look at the most common mistakes of beginners and how they can be avoided. And at the same time, we'll talk about which group of people most often encounters certain problems with keto nutrition and why.

## Mistake number one

Often low carb high protein and fat diets are promoted by athletes to boost physical performance. Depending on the sport or any physical task, the keto diet can have a different effect. Athletes usually follow diets under the supervision of an experienced nutritionist who closely monitors the athlete's body condition and sports results. This means that the dosages and the ratio of proteins, fats, and carbohydrates are selected very individually, they are constantly regulated and a strict nutrition plan is drawn up.

Research has shown that sports that require high intensity within a short duration, a decrease in performance was found. In anaerobic and even some aerobic sports requiring a short burst of intense energy; players and athletes are not advised to follow a diet such as a keto. But since ketone is a better fuel option for the heart and it increases mental focuses significantly; it can be equally helpful for other sports such as swimming and running.

Looking at athletes observing keto, many make the first very widespread mistake: is not understanding that keto isn't the same for everyone. Depending on your body health, metabolism and lifestyle as well as the intensity of physical activity it can be determined whether keto is the right approach to follow.

The question is how do athletes maintain keto? If one of the athletes inspires you to practice keto, you should remember that the goals that athletes set for themselves, adhering to a particular type of diet, are often far from the desire to be healthy. In most cases, nutrition for a professional athlete is a way to prepare the body for a sports result. There are many reasons and mistakes that athletes make when following keto which can cause negative side effects. Athletes can suffer from severe nutritional deficiencies that can become quite dangerous when combined with high athletic performance.

## Mistake number two

One of the biggest fears that athletes face when following keto is assuming that they are consuming too much fat. This misconception is caused by adding large quantities of fat into daily meals. But on the other hand that's how keto works, meals consist of almost 80% fat of daily calorie intake. So it's quite normal to be eating more fat while on the diet. A quick example on the fat quantity you're supposed to be taking on the diet; your daily fat intake for an athlete who consumes around 2900 calories that is equivalent to 256g of fat that your body needs to be in a proper ketosis state. Many athletes think of fat as an enemy and end uploading their bodies with carbs before a workout for muscle gain. Understanding how keto really works is the right way to get the most out of it.

Therefore, if you decide on keto, you will have to stop considering fats as your enemy.

## Mistake number three

Another mistake when switching to keto nutrition is the desire to load your body with a large amount of protein. Athletes do this to build muscle. Other people may make this mistake trying to replace the missing amount of carbohydrates.

This is not true! Excessive protein intake can cause health problems, such as gluconeogenesis, which turns amino acids back into glucose, thus reversing ketosis. Many low-fat diets should include a lot of protein and little fat. But here it's the opposite! Keto is high in fat with adequate protein intake. Do not get involved in protein foods. Keto's diet allows only moderate protein.

## Mistake number four

Hidden carbohydrates: Even by limiting carbohydrate intake, we are usually fooled by other ingredients that are not considered carbohydrates that we did not know about. Carbohydrates do not necessarily mean only bread, pasta, and rice. Hidden carbohydrates can be found in processed foods, dairy alternatives that contain sugar because sugar is considered a carbohydrate, and even some types of fruits and vegetables are "starchy," which leads to carbohydrates. They have the ability to accumulate and, thus, increase glucose levels. Other non-obvious carbohydrates, such as salad dressings and sauces containing sugar or other types of sweeteners, such as honey.

Find out more about what products and ingredients to write down on your next shopping list on page 50.

## Mistake number five

The next mistake is by far the most common one. The initial side effects of keto can be difficult and unfortunately many take a short way and just quit. This takes place in the first few days as the metabolic change takes place. Your body needs a little time to readjust its settings. Patience is key to the success of keto and it's important to conduct it correctly. You must understand that when you enter ketosis state every single cell in the body must switch to using fat instead of glucose for energy. That isn't something that can be achieved overnight and certainly isn't easy. At this point, insulin levels drop which causes the body to lose water and sodium. That is why it's critical to make up for the lost water and sodium by staying well hydrated and adding enough sodium in your diet to prevent side effects such as 'keto flu'. The best thing for anyone who is progressing quickly into keto is to be patient and strong. Do not let initial side effects such as nausea and dizziness control you. Be strong and stay hydrated and eat well. It's only a matter of days before your body adjusts to the new system and then you'll feel stronger and fitter than before.

Many who start any diet, including keto, eat the same

monotonous food.



## Mistake number six

Some can get carried away a little bit by over-controlling their food. This problem can be caused by many reasons but the most common one is social pressure. Yes we all know are living in quite a competitive world. Society imposes certain stereotypes on food, appearance, how we should look, how much to weigh, what to wear and with whom to communicate. We have to be the best level and this adds pressure on our mental health by everyone around us. That is why it is best to start keto or implement any significant change in your lifestyle or diet when you are on holiday. Making a major turn in your lifestyle in the midst of the busy rhythm of life is a really bad idea. You will stress yourself and won't be allowing your body to fully adjust to the change. It's important to understand your body and give it enough time to cope with change, you must also never ignore the warning signs. Our bodies are like machines when something is wrong, it indicates it. Don't ignore these signs. Don't stick to a meal plan that isn't right for your body. Make some amendments to adjust your schedule while staying on the diet. Always listen to your body!

# Mistakes that are common to different groups of people who start keto



For many diabetics, keto might be the right diet and lifestyle for them, but just like other people, diabetics will face side effects by following keto. Although keto might work for people with diabetes type 2 by lowering glucose levels in the blood while staying healthy. One of the most common mistake diabetics makes when following keto is assuming that such a diet is best for everyone. That is not entirely true. No diet comes in an all-in-one package that is fit for all types of bodies and diseases. It is very important to individualize the diet to meet your special needs. Not all bodies are the same and not everybody reacts the same way to significant changes brought by the diet.

Most people who suffer from diabetes focus on what's off the limits instead of paying attention to what should they really eat. As human beings, we don't cope well with starvation or any type of strictly restricted diet full of deprivation and dull rabbit food- unless you have an iron-willpower but even then you wouldn't last long. It's a natural response from our bodies! On the other hand, people with diabetes must balance their blood sugar, and this is a vital necessity for them. One way or another, you have to find a healthy compromise in order to keep your body healthy.

What happens when someone with diabetes starts the keto diet? First thing is that you would have to restrict your carbohydrates intake to 5% of your daily intake. That can be a huge decrease for those who are used to eating pasta, rice, and bread. Again, we all have different lifestyles so some of us might find this step easy to follow while others will experience deprivation and uncontrollable cravings for carbs. By lowering your carbohydrate intake, you will need to adjust your insulin dose. Of course, make sure to consult your doctor first. This step is important when you first enter keto, to help you control the highs.

Type 1 diabetes patients can experience negative side effects such as diabetic ketoacidosis which is a life-threatening condition. Another mistake can be missing your insulin shot while you are in ketosis, this can cause sickness. Another thing to keep in mind if you have diabetes is that some may find that following the keto diet can increase insulin resistance which then might contribute to causing type 2 diabetes. Also, dairy products can have side effects such as causing a spike in blood sugar levels. **It is critical to have a doctor follow up with you when you being keto diet because any short-term low carb strict diet must be carefully monitored for diabetes patients.** There is an increased risk of hypoglycemia in type 2 diabetes patients in the result of following a restricted carb diet plan.

Also, it is important to take proper supplements and vitamins that you may deprive of when following keto such as Vitamin D. It is best to take vitamin supplements and have your doctor follow up.

What is the one popular reason that makes people want to start a diet? Weight loss or weight gain. That's right, many start diets in order to lose excess weight or to try to gain some.

Keto, such as other popular diets, promise weight loss and a healthier lifestyle for those seeking, especially people who suffer from overweight. In addition to the mistakes that we have already described, people who want to lose weight make a few more mistakes. What are these errors?

When starting a low carb diet such as keto, many assume that I can eat more food and still lose weight because it's not carbs! This is not entirely true. At the first stage, indeed the amount of food consumed increases, just out of habit. But, after some time, we begin to feel hunger less often and saturate faster. This is because with keto nutrition, fats, not carbohydrates, are our source of energy. Fat is an ideal fuel for our body. It takes more time to recycle it. Our body spends more energy on this, and yet, the feeling of fullness lasts much longer than after consuming carbohydrates. Moreover, in the cold season, the use of fats gives more heat in our body. This means that you will warm up faster and freeze less.

Nevertheless, if your goal is to lose weight, it is better if you control the amount of food consumed.

It was previously believed that the main cause of obesity is overeating and lack of exercise. Of course, this has some common sense, but the problem of excess weight is more associated with metabolic disorders in our body. Modern food has a large bias towards carbohydrates, rejection of fats and offers insufficient quality protein. Agree that our body is unlikely to become healthier if we eat potato chips with beef flavor. Moreover, we voluntarily deceive ourselves. Our brain thinks that it eats meat, because it has analyzed the smell and taste of meat, and our body, digesting starch, shouts to our brain: we need protein! Give at least a serving of protein! It is this situation that gives rise to a constant feeling of unsatisfied hunger. That's why diets such as keto are designed to give us the most needed in sufficient amounts to help us solve overweight problems.

So, those who lose weight are faced with additional difficulties. As you know keto works only when you really stick to it which means no cheat meals, no open meals, no binge eating. Any change of track will lead you back to your starting point, straight out of ketosis mode. Frequent snacks for keto are unacceptable. For many, this is a purely psychological problem. But it needs to be solved, otherwise, the result from the keto will be zero. Especially since sometimes people mistake 'low-carb' snacks as 'zero carbs treat' and end up overeating of them throughout the day which not only adds up your total calorie intake but also increases that amount of carbs consumed which can throw you out of ketosis mode and you are back to start point.

Another psychological problem is the fear of fats. We already wrote about this, but overweight people have a very stable bias against fat. As soon as they begin keto diet they will assume that no more carbs are allowed and focus on protein and a little fat. But keto doesn't work without consuming a high percentage of fats in your meals because you are not supplying your body with enough glucose anymore for energy so in return it switched to burning fat instead. So not consuming enough fats is one serious mistake that many overweight people tend to make.

It is also not worth replacing fats with proteins. This type of nutrition corresponds to other popular diets and it requires compliance with some other rules. High protein intake and little fat will not put your body into ketosis mode and you might end up with health issues because we can't survive on just protein. Our bodies need less refined sugar, white flour, and more fiber, vitamins, and minerals. So don't be afraid of eating more fat, just make sure you calculate exactly how much your body needs to ensure that you are properly following the keto diet.

We should also talk about salt intake. We all know to much salt intake causes weight gain due to water retention in our body. But once you start the keto diet, your salt intake will drastically decrease because you are not consuming processed and refined food anymore. But that doesn't mean that it should stay that way. Our body needs a percentage of sodium in our diet. Many are oblivious to the fact that when you're on keto, you need to take in more sodium. Salt is simply necessary so that a sufficient amount of gastric juice is secreted, which in turn is necessary for all enzymes to work properly. Therefore, do not exclude salt from your diet, and if you notice that its intake has been greatly reduced, add it to your water. A great solution maybe if you put a few crystals of coarse sea salt under your tongue. This should be done immediately after eating, especially protein. In general, you need to experiment a little and choose the option that is right for you.

The most important thing to keep in mind when you suffer from obesity is that the numbers on the scale may not drop much when you are in ketosis, but that doesn't mean you are not losing fat. Your body measurements might change while your weight might only fluctuate a little. This often affects most overweight people, making them go impatient when following the diet. Practice shows that during the two weeks of the diet, one week is spent on the fact that kilograms are lost, but this often does not affect the volume. But in the second week, there is an active loss of volumes, but the arrow on the scales practically does not move. This also depends on your metabolism, not everyone is the same. Some may lose a few pounds per month, while others will take 2 weeks. Some studies have shown that there could be a slight increase in metabolism during the initial stages of ketosis which slowly fades off within the first month. Because metabolism depends on body weight which in return decreases when water is lost by following a low-carb diet.

Sometimes overweights are too consumed with fear that they are eating too much, which leads them to practically starving themselves. This is not how keto works at all! Calories are calories and you are required to consume a specific amount depending on your body needs and lifestyle. Anything above or below that amount will have negative side effects and can put you through serious illness and diseases. At the beginning of the book, we already talked about the fact that on the keto diet in our body, similar processes are launched as during a hunger strike. This is the production of ketone bodies. But unlike hunger, we get energy for life. It is very important! Therefore, do not starve to strengthen the action of keto. Moreover, our metabolism works on the principle of the firebox. The more firewood we throw at it, the more heat it gives out and the faster all the fuel burns. If nothing is toss into the furnace, then the fire in the firebox will go out and the system will not work. So is our metabolism - so that it burns all the "fuel" consumed by us, we must eat regularly.

One more thing that not just overweight people must keep in mind, make sure you drink enough water.

This is crucially important for everyone whether they are following the keto diet or not. Not drinking enough water is one significant mistake that many make and it can ruin any plans of weight loss that you have in mind. Just think, about 50 ounces of fluid is needed only by our intestines. About the same as our kidneys remove toxins from the body. As well as other organs, skin, epithelial tissues ... This does not mean that you need to drink water in barrels, but make sure that you consume the recommended water level daily. The average amount of water you need to drink daily is based on your body weight, 1 ounce of water to every pound of bodyweight.

Another mistake regarding meals is taking your meals while you're watching TV or using your phone. Mindless eating is on the contributing factors of weight gain and overconsumption. When you don't focus on your food and end up eating too quickly while you're being distracted. It could be hard for you to feel full. You might eat an entire meal while watching the TV closely but by the time you' are finished with it; you find yourself still hungry. The best solution to this problem is to take your meals in the kitchen or anywhere away from such distractions and just focus on your meal. Enjoy it and chew slowly, you'll find yourself full and happy.

Another major lifestyle mistake people make while following keto is that they don't get enough sleep. Anywhere from 6-8 hours per nights. That could be hard to maintain by students but it's critically important. Sleeping enough every night allow the body enough time to rest, recharge itself and to enable it to function properly the next day. Lack of sleep causes fatigue, weakness and sometimes headaches and dizziness especially when you're on keto.

## Keto for lifestyle. Possible problems

You might think that only overweight people start going on diets. This is not true. But even regular healthy people might go on diets simply for 'healthier' lifestyle. But sometimes we are misled about what a really healthy lifestyle should look like. This does not mean that you should overwork yourself in the gym for hours and there is an only salad. Some people can eat "healthy food", but their lifestyle and daily routine are completely opposite, which, in turn, gives no results at all. When it comes to keto, it's often easier for people who are fit and healthy to follow it and keep up. Because they lead an active life with a balanced calorie consumption throughout the day. But everyone makes mistakes right? So how could a healthy person make mistakes by being healthy while following the keto diet?

The first mistake these people make is that they aren't mentally prepared to take on the challenge of keto. For a diet like a keto to work, almost 95% success is mental. The human brain can trigger hormones and send signals to different parts of the body to function. So for keto to work on you, your brain must be prepared to handle it. Now you must wonder how can someone prep their brain for such a thing? The first step, the most important initial step in anything, is to carefully plan your routine. Part of that requires you to plan your meals and at this point, where many make their second biggest mistake. Without a meal plan and preparation, it could be extremely difficult for you to keep up with keto. If you were used to eating a lot of snacking throughout the day. You will find yourself walking to the fridge every two hours unconsciously that's because your brain has gotten used to the old habits of eating every two hours so it's sending the signal to your body to go to the fridge and grab a snack.

How can we fix this problem?

Meal plan and preparation. When you plan your meals by time, you are mentally preparing yourself to follow the plan and block any thoughts or signals that encourage you to snack or eat when you're not really hungry. We often get confused between are we really hungry or should I just drink water?

The next mistake is very common among students and people with tight work schedules throughout the day; stress. Stress is something many of us face and some only experience it temporarily during difficult times and others live with it. For students, stress levels may rise significantly during exams weeks and this can cause negative side effects on the body. Some people are known to lose weight when they are overstressed, that is caused by loss of appetite mostly. They would much less than they normally consume and by overthinking and planning they are burning more energy because their brains are processing to fast. But for other people, stress can contribute to mindless and comfort food eating. This leads to binge eating and overconsumption of calories which in return leads to great weight gain. So how can this issue be fixed? It may be hard for some people and easy for others but stress doesn't just affect our mood. It raises cortisol levels which in return increases blood sugar levels. What happened next is that with the raise blood sugar levels the brain sends out signals to are-charge the glycogen levels in the body so that it can process fast. That's when we start craving carbohydrates. So you must know that is is very important to manage your stress of you experience any.

One of the best ways to manage stress and also a mistake many make is exercising. People who don't exercise or don't exercise enough while following a keto diet will not be seeing positive results in their weight loss goals. The average time duration for exercise can range from 25-30 minutes daily. However, exhausting training in the gym is not the best solution. It is better to choose a good qigong gymnastics, yoga or something similar. If for some reason you cannot work out, find another way to relieve stress. It can be reading, drawing, walking or gardening.

You must understand that managing your time, stress, meal planning and preparation and getting enough sleep are the key to the success of keto. Without these factors, you will not reach your goal and you will only experience the negative side effects of keto.

## How to start and not give up right away

### Adaptation time

We all know that nothing worth having ever comes easy to us but how hard could it be? With all the promises that keto offers, from a healthier body to losing excess weight and improved mental and physical performance. How do we get there?

When starting keto you must understand the stages you will have to get through in order to reach the stage where you can continue with the diet that's when you're the body has fully adjusted. But unfortunately, many people neglect this fact and just give up in the first few weeks sometimes assuming that they failed to do it right or it's not working out for them and probably made their lives worse.

Jumping into ketosis is the first step you make that's when you are changing your body state from relying on carbohydrates and start producing ketones as an alternative energy source. This is called establishing nutritional ketosis, you' are depleting your liver from glycogen. This state doesn't happen overnight, it usually takes anywhere from one to 3 weeks depending on your body. This might be physically exhausting for you. You are not doing it wrong, this is completely normal. The reason the physical exhaustion happens is that your muscles aren't prepared to utilize ketones for energy yet.

Athletes and overactive people who have intense workout

schedules during the initial stages of keto it is essential to take it a little easy on your workouts. Try not to exceed 30 minutes of intense cardio or resistance workouts because it requires a lot of muscle strength and energy. This will be hard to achieve because your muscles are ready just yet. So don't over-work yourself out in the gym during the first week of starting keto. You will be able to tackle it all once you are in full ketosis mode. Patience is key.

It is very important when observing keto not to starve, especially at the beginning. You must remember that keto is not a starvation diet! It doesn't work out if you starve yourself or eat less than your daily calorie requirements. The key to solving this problem by managing your meals. Early preparation of meals leaves you organized even during your busy schedule. You can plan your meals and prepare them all in one day and keep them in containers in the fridge. That way when you don't have the time to make a keto meal, it will be ready for pick up. This step is very important and it will be discussed more deeply later in this book. Being prepared and setting a meal schedule for yourself prevents binge eating, snacking and keeps you full and energized throughout the day. It also makes adapting to keto a lot easier where you wouldn't have to suffer from debating what to cook every day. Therefore, make sure that you eat enough, not too little and not too much, but enough for the needs of your body.

If you are starving, then you are sure to abandon the diet, regardless of how useful it is for you. Stay concentrated and don't neglect your body! Eat well and stay balanced, that's the best way to tackle the difficult initial adaptation period so later on, you will start noticing the significant results of the keto diet.

The next mistake people seem to make when adapting to keto is not drinking enough water. This means that they either drink too little or to much water, both can throw you off balance a little bit. Here's why; when you don't drink enough water your body will enter dehydration state because with the produced ketones you will lose all your water weight, thus leaving the body completely dehydrated. On the other hand, when you drink to much water, you are losing sodium. That's why in keto you are supposed to make sure you consume enough sodium.

Be sure to consult your doctor to help you determine the amount of water you need to drink daily.

## Lack of minerals

During keto or any other special diet, you will be facing some minor side effects that can be fixed in order to follow the diet properly and remain healthy. Because what good would it be if you lose excess weight but suffered from a long list of nutritional deficiencies.half of the loose weight is usually water weight not fat weight. With keto, your body will be running low of minerals such as sodium, magnesium, potassium, and calcium. This is another common assumption; just because you start running low on these minerals doesn't mean you can't back up for the loss! The replacement won't be in medicines or any funny remedies, instead it's available right in the ingredients you will be using in your keto meal plan.

First let's begin with sodium, during ketosis you will lose water weight, thus losing sodium as well. The sodium loss is even greater for people visiting the gym because of their intense and active lifestyle routine. One of the most common ways sodium leaves the body is through sweat and urine. But that doesn't necessarily mean that everyone on the diet will be suffering from low sodium levels. In fact, overweight people are often consuming too much sodium which traps the water in, raising the scale higher with the water weight. It's true that keto allows us to burn the stored fat in our bodies but when it comes to nutrients like sodium, we don't have any backup reserves because it's found in the bloodstream. So once we lose too much of it, we need to replace. It is advised to run blood tests to check which nutrients do you suffer a deficiency from. Often the symptoms for low sodium levels include weakness, fatigue, and dizziness. These same symptoms accompany the phase of "keto-flu", which usually happens at the very beginning of the diet. Therefore, it is better to periodically conduct tests to be completely sure.

As for magnesium, it's been shown that magnesium helps to calm the brain down and relieve from muscle cramps. You might be wondering now what is really lowering minerals levels in our bodies during ketosis? Like we said sodium is lost when you are losing to much water weight but other lifestyle habits and activities can contribute to lower magnesium levels. Such activities include intense physical workout, lack of sleep and of course stress. The good news is just like with sodium, you don't need drugs to balance it. Great sources of magnesium mostly come from animal protein. Magnesium is also found in leafy greens such as spinach and other fruits such as avocado.

Because keto is low on dairy products, many develop a calcium deficiency. What many people don't seem to know is calcium is not only found in the regular cup of milk we are told to drink since we were young; other low-carb ingredients are high in calcium such as aged cheese. It is important to keep an eye on calcium level because as we get older, as it declines in the bone tissue. The tricky part is figuring out whether you were suffering from calcium deficiency or not. There are symptoms that you can be experiencing that will indicate calcium deficiency such as dental issues, irritability, and muscle cramps. But these symptoms might only appear in the long-term, so it is advised to take blood tests regularly to make sure you don't suffer from any mineral deficiency.

## Do not reduce fat

One of the reasons keto fails for many people is by not consuming enough fat. This book highlights this point repeatedly because it's one big mistake that breaks down into multiple mistakes that not only fail the keto experience for you but also cause health issues such as thyroid and metabolic disorders.

When you're starting keto and drastically reducing carbs intake, it might be difficult to eat fat. You must understand that if you consume about 2000 calories a day, on keto you still need those 2000 calories which will consist of 80% fat, that's around 170g of fat.

However, that doesn't mean that you can binge eat on bacon all you want. The good thing about fat is that it's very satiating. So eating the right amount will not only satisfy your calorie requirements, but it will also fill you up and leave you feeling full for a longer time. The correct approach to consuming enough fat is by figuring out exactly how many grams your body needs. Your next step is adjusting your fat sources. You must remember that fat is what you will be eating the most so you have to make sure it provides your body with energy throughout the day. The best fat sources are healthy oils like avocado and coconut oil.

## The challenge

What makes a challenge so encouraging or frightening? It's never easy. Everyone might have a different experience in a challenge but it's never to easy for anyone to follow. When it comes to keto, it is a real challenge that not only changes your lifestyle but your entire body system. The transition period can be not only difficult but depressing, dreadful and exhausting. It could be the reason to quitting or motivation for those who enjoy a hard challenge. But why does it sound so dreading? Is there any way to make it easier? The answer is yes, by avoiding these common mistakes people usually make during their initial week on keto. Preventing these mistakes will not only make starting keto easier, but it will also widen your knowledge about how your body works, thus helping you understand it more.

The first mistake is thinking: what have I gotten myself into?

This is broken down too different aspects, mainly it's about what you force yourself to eat. As human beings, we don't get pleased by eating the same food every single day, unless it was our favorite! And what is the first assumption people make when starting a diet? I can't eat anything other than dull colorless lettuce salad and drink lots of water. This is not a diet, it's basically another term for starvation. This will drain your energy, you might still lose a few pounds but the chance that you'll quit and binge eat on anything 'unhealthy' is high. If you starve yourself, you don't have enough fat, and you simply don't have enough energy. You will end up with a craving to eat and, as a rule, go to the nearest donut shop. But why is this happening? The answer is that you are not just starving in your body, your brain is telling you that if you cannot eat anything, then you are starving.

Be sure to plan your menus and in the first week, it is better not to rely on self-research. To follow keto correctly, you need an accurate calculation of your daily calorie needs depending on your body and lifestyle. This step not only ensures that your body remains healthy but also ensures that the transition period is easier and more stable. In a week or so, you'll get comfortable and you will no longer need to follow a strict plan in everything, but at first, it's better not to rely on yourself.

Be sure to plan your menus and in the first week, it is better not to rely on self-research. To follow keto correctly, you need an accurate calculation of your daily calorie needs depending on your body and lifestyle. This step not only ensures that your body remains healthy but also ensures that the transition period is easier and more stable.

In a week or so, you'll get comfortable and you will no longer need to follow a strict plan in everything, but at first, it's better not to rely on yourself.

Staying away from unnecessary carbs on an extremely low carb diet sounds easy, right? In fact, it's not at all. Just because you aren't enjoying your favorite pasta or rice dish doesn't mean you aren't consuming too many carbs. Carbs are very sneaky, they can be found inside the least suspecting ingredients. When following any low-carb diet or anything that targets weight loss, eating hidden carbs will obviously prevent you from losing weight and you are most likely to gain extra weight. But on keto consuming more than the required amount of carbs, around 5%, will throw you out of ketosis mode. You have then left with the option of either starting again, or continuing keto 'on your rules' which isn't real keto at all or simply giving up.

How to avoid this problem? Study food! This doesn't mean you have to become a nutritionist. Thanks to the internet and books, it has become a lot easier to check and research such information. So here is a time-saver for you, these are the most common sneaky carbs people consume unintentionally.

One of the most cunning ways companies sell their products is by marketing them under the name 'healthy' or 'light'. Examples include fizzy drinks, energy drinks, granola bars, fiber cereals even those marked as 'sugar-free'. Even in the dairy section where you might be picking up some 'low-fat healthy' plain yogurt, you might be surprised to know it can contain up to 30g of carbs!

So how to avoid these hidden carbs? Read the nutrition label!

Check the amount of sugar and carbs in each item. Don't be fooled by marketing names that target people who are too lazy to read the label.

Think about what is inside the products that have been peeled, fat-free, incredibly processed, packaged in a beautiful bag that says "Healthy Food"? I think the answer is obvious.

# Part 3.
# Let's get started!

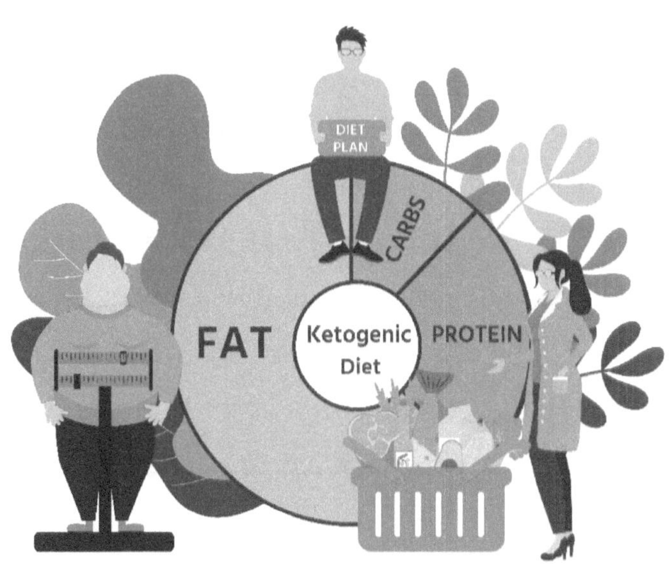

# Cleansing

When you are well into a diet and progressing well and on one calm evening you start craving double chocolate peanut cookies which are sitting in the cookie jar in your kitchen. It's going to take strong will power and a good distraction to get that bad idea out of your head for good.

That's one mistake we all seem to make. But with keto, it's different because while other diets might promote 'cheat days' or 'cheat meals' every once in a while; keto has no tolerance for cheating. It's a lifestyle, a long-term sustainable diet that can be canceled the minute you break the rule.

The best way to ensure you stick to keto and prevent such incidents to happen is by cleansing your house of the restricted ingredients.

Simply get rid out of it, all those unhealthy treats, high sugar beverages, and candy bars; give it all away. The next step is to restock your kitchen with the right food. Then you can make your own keto-friendly treats and snacks which you can enjoy without feeling guilty and while staying in ketosis. Find out more about what food should be on your next grocery list and what needs to leave your kitchen right now on page 50.

# Adjusting

After you' are done with restocking your kitchen with the appropriate ingredients it's time to avoid the next mistake and start adjusting your grain and dairy consumption.

You might be wondering why specifically grain and milk that requires adjusting. Here's why.

Whole grains are packed with fiber and aids digestion, it is also high in carbohydrates. Keto practically forbids grains on the diet because a small amount can throw you out of ketosis especially if you add up the sneaky carbs you consume throughout the day.

As for milk, while one cup of full-fat milk is packed with essential minerals and vitamins such as calcium, potassium, vitamins A, D and B12, and other nutrients. But just like grains, it contains a lot of carbs and sugar. You can still drink full-fat milk but you will be on the risk of canceling ketosis if you weren't very careful. On the other hand, there are other substitutes for low carb milk that you can have instead of regular milk. That way, you aren't depriving yourself nor are you throwing your body out of ketosis and back too starting point.

### Healthy fats

It's true that you should be eating a lot of fat on keto since it makes up almost 80% of your daily meals. But you must understand that not all fats are the same and certainly you shouldn't be eating all of them.

Types of bad fats include:

- Processed polyunsaturated fats and processed trans fat. These fats are found not only in 'processed' food but also in vegetables and seeds such as canola, corn, peanuts, soybean, and sunflower.

- Processed trans fat is found in 'processed' food such as margarine, fast food, and store-bought bakes.

- Now let's take a look at the healthy fats we should be focusing on;

- Natural polyunsaturated fats which are high in omega 3, are found in seeds like chia, flaxseed and of course fish.

- Monounsaturated fats are found in nut oils like macadamia, avocado, and extra-virgin olive oil. It increases insulin resistance and decreases blood pressure.

- Natural fat is found in dairy products and meat from animals that were grass-fed.

- Saturated fats include eggs, cream, butter, ghee, and coconut oil. It helps prevent risks of heart disease in the future. It also removes cholesterol out of your blood system.

## Protein

With the high fat, low carb intake you need moderate consumption of protein to balance it out. Obvious protein sources include red meat, eggs and vegetables such as broccoli. But you can also incorporate other forms of protein such as using protein powders. This is usually done by athletes or bodybuilders who have larger muscle mass for intense physical performance. However the problem lies in the amount of protein that you are required to take. This is where mistakes happen. Again, not everybody is the same therefore it is critical that keto is not based on assumptions and self-research, you need practical measurements and tests to determine how much protein your body needs. If you spend all day working at the office, your body obviously won't be needing as much protein as a boxer or a football player. Average protein recommendation is around 1.7g per kg  of your total body weight. But for people who suffer from health issues and diseases such as cancer they may have too decrease too just 1g per kg of body weight,

Great examples of high protein food are eggs, salmon, string cheese, milk. Shrimp and chicken thighs.

## Carbs

It's true that keto restricts carbs intake to a very low level but that doesn't mean it's less important than fats and protein. It plays an important role as well in sustaining ketosis.

While almost all the food we consume is packed with carbs and sugar even those 'healthy' options. You might be faced with a serious problem in not knowing where to get your carbs from? To solve the dilemma, here are some of the best low-carb ingredients to add to your grocery list:

- Bell peppers- high in vitamins C and A plus they are inflammatory.
- Broccoli- the superfood that not only packed with vitamins C and K, but also decreases insulin resistance.
- Zucchini- the healthier option for regular spaghetti. It's not just great as a 'zoodle' dish but also packed with vitamin C.
- Spinach- provides protection for the heart and eye.
- Cauliflower- not only helps to prevent cancer, but it's also packed with vitamin C.
- Cucumber- it's refreshing, aids brain health and one cup has only 4g of carbs.
- Tomatoes- not just green vegetables are great high-carb substitutes. Packed with potassium and vitamins.

Water

The only element that we can't survive long without, it's what keeps our bodies running and functioning. That's why our bodies are made of 70% water. Water cleanses the body, helps the flow of blood, regulates the kidneys and basically manages everything else in the body. Many people don't understand the importance of water and often neglect the fact that we are drinking a lot less water than our bodies need.

The problem is, not drinking enough water not only creates digestive and kidney issues but also aids weight gain and makes weight loss seem impossible.

So remember to drink at least 2.5 or 3 liters of water every day.

Lack of water dries the skin, therefore, allowing acne and dark spots and wrinkles too attack the skin. It can also lead to major health difficulties caused by food blockage in the intestines due to lack of water,

So you must manage your water intake and make sure you are not drinking less than 2.5 liters a day to ensure a healthier body and a better life.

# GUIDE

After reading about all those mistakes beginners make when starting keto it's now time to take a look at the three categories that food is divided into. This guide will help you stay away from the restricted food.

## Unlimited access

Foods that you can eat without restrictions are mostly low-carb vegetables that are packed with vitamins and nutrients.

- Asparagus-contains fiber nutrients
- Cabbage- high sulfur percentage, contains probiotic fiber
- Broccoli- omega-3 and vitamins
- Kale- Omega-3, fiber nutrients
- Celery- high fiber
- Cucumber- contains cucurbitacin E
- Brussels sprouts- provides 80% of the recommended daily intake of vitamin C
- Chard

- Olives
- Radish
- Collards
- Bok choy
- Avocado
- Lettuce
- Mineral water
- Green tea
- Bulletproof coffee
- Cinnamon

# Limited

Foods that can be consumed in limited quantities.

- Full-fat milk
- Strawberries
- Coconut
- Raspberries
- Blackberries
- Plums
- Blueberries
- Olive oil
- Pastured chicken/turkey
- Artichokes
- Eggplant
- Turnip
- Green beans
- Onion
- Sweet potato
- rhubarb
- Winter squash
- Raw almonds
- Almond flour
- Coconut flour
- Pecans

- Cashews
- Hazelnuts
- Non-organic butter or ghee
- Herbal tea
- Stevia
- Monk fruit

# Banned

Banned food on keto

- Root vegetables- potato, carrots, beets, etc...
- Grains such- cereals, bread, oatmeal, popcorn, etc...
- Starches- pasta, rice, quinoa, barley, bulgar,
- Sweets- Candy, cookies, puddings, cakes, etc...
- sweeteners - honey, agave, nectar, maple syrup, etc...
- Legumes- beans of all kind, lentils, chickpeas
- Alcohol- every single type
- Low-fat dairy- anything that's fat-free or low-fat in the dairy section
- Dips and sauces- ketchup, BBQ sauce, tomato sauce
- Sweetened drinks- soda, juice, milkshakes, smoothies,
- Fruits- watermelon, apples, pear, banana, plums, grapefruit, mango, etc...

---

*Thanks for reading! Please add a short review on Amazon and let me know what you thought!*

Thanks and good luck!
**Tina Lee**

www.ingramcontent.com/pod-product-compliance
Lightning Source LLC
Chambersburg PA
CBHW051123250726
48655CB00007B/2849